Probiotics Health Treatment Guide for Beginners

Benefits of Probiotics and Digestive Health

By

Dalton Nathaniel

Copyright@2023

Table of Contents

CHAPTER 1

Introduction to Probiotics

1.1 What is Probiotics

Probiotics are living microorganisms that provide health benefits when consumed in adequate amounts. These beneficial bacteria and yeasts, mostly from the Lactobacillus and Bifidobacterium genera, play a crucial role in maintaining a balanced gut microbiome. The term "probiotic" is derived from Greek words "pro," meaning "promoting," and "biotic," meaning "life," emphasizing their function in supporting good health.

Probiotics can be found naturally in various fermented foods such as yogurt, kefir, sauerkraut, kimchi, and certain cheeses. Additionally, they are available in the form of dietary supplements, which offer specific strains in concentrated doses.

1.2 The Role of Probiotics in Gut Health

The gut, or gastrointestinal tract, is a complex ecosystem populated by trillions of microorganisms, collectively known as the gut microbiota. This diverse community of bacteria, viruses, and fungi plays a crucial role in maintaining digestive health, regulating the immune system, synthesizing certain vitamins, and protecting against harmful pathogens.

Probiotics contribute significantly to the balance and functionality of the gut microbiome. They help by:

1. Restoring Microbial Balance: The gut microbiota can be influenced by factors such as diet, stress, medications (like antibiotics), and lifestyle choices. These factors can disrupt the delicate balance of beneficial and harmful bacteria in the gut. Probiotics help restore this balance by promoting the growth of beneficial bacteria and inhibiting the growth of harmful ones.

2. Enhancing Digestion: Probiotics aid in the breakdown and absorption of nutrients, particularly in the small intestine. They produce enzymes that break down complex carbohydrates and

fibers, making them easier for the body to digest and utilize.

3. Strengthening the Gut Barrier: The gut lining acts as a barrier, preventing harmful substances and pathogens from entering the bloodstream. Probiotics play a role in enhancing the integrity of this barrier, reducing the risk of leaky gut syndrome, which can lead to inflammation and various health issues.

4. Modulating the Immune System: Approximately 70-80% of the body's immune system resides in the gut-associated lymphoid tissue (GALT). Probiotics interact with immune cells in the GALT, promoting a balanced immune response. They can help reduce excessive inflammation and

strengthen the body's defense
against infections and diseases.

5. Producing Beneficial Compounds:
   Certain strains of probiotics can
   produce short-chain fatty acids
   (SCFAs), such as butyrate, acetate,
   and propionate. These SCFAs
   provide energy for the cells lining
   the colon, support a healthy pH
   environment in the gut, and have
   anti-inflammatory effects.

1.3 Benefits of Probiotics for Overall Health

Beyond their influence on gut health,
probiotics have been associated with a
range of other health benefits,
affecting various aspects of overall
well-being. Some of these benefits
include:

1. Improved Digestive Function:
   Probiotics can help alleviate
   common digestive issues such as
   bloating, gas, and constipation.
   They aid in maintaining a healthy
   balance of gut bacteria, which can
   lead to better digestion and
   nutrient absorption.

2. Enhanced Immune Function: By
   supporting a balanced immune
   response, probiotics may help
   reduce the severity and duration of
   common infections, such as the
   common cold, as well as
   potentially supporting immune
   function in individuals with
   autoimmune conditions.

3. Management of Irritable Bowel
   Syndrome (IBS): IBS is a chronic
   gastrointestinal disorder
   characterized by abdominal pain,
   bloating, and changes in bowel

habits. Some studies suggest that certain probiotic strains may help alleviate symptoms and improve the quality of life in individuals with IBS.

4. Mental Health and Cognitive Function: The gut-brain axis is a bidirectional communication system between the gut and the brain. Emerging research indicates that probiotics may have a positive impact on mental health by influencing the gut-brain axis, potentially reducing symptoms of anxiety, depression, and stress.

5. Cardiovascular Health: Some studies suggest that specific probiotics may have a modest positive effect on reducing blood pressure and lowering LDL cholesterol levels, contributing to improved cardiovascular health.

6. Skin Health: The balance of gut bacteria can influence skin health and conditions like acne and eczema. Probiotics may help improve certain skin conditions by promoting a balanced gut microbiome and reducing inflammation.

7. Allergy Management: Probiotics may play a role in modulating the immune response, potentially reducing the severity of allergic reactions and managing conditions like eczema and allergic rhinitis.

8. Weight Management: Some research indicates that probiotics might contribute to weight loss and support healthy weight management by influencing gut bacteria associated with metabolism.

It's important to note that while probiotics offer numerous potential health benefits, individual responses may vary. Furthermore, the effectiveness of probiotics depends on factors such as the specific strains used, the dosage, and the individual's overall health and lifestyle. Before starting any probiotic supplementation, it is advisable to consult a healthcare professional, especially for individuals with underlying health conditions or compromised immune systems.

CHAPTER 2

Understanding Gut Health

2.1 The Gut Microbiome: An Overview

The gut microbiome refers to the vast and diverse community of microorganisms that reside in the gastrointestinal tract. It is a complex ecosystem comprising bacteria, viruses, fungi, and other microorganisms that play a fundamental role in maintaining overall health. The gut microbiome is unique to each individual, influenced by various factors such as genetics, diet, environment, and lifestyle.

Key points about the gut microbiome:

- Diversity: The gut microbiome is incredibly diverse, with thousands of different microbial species. This diversity is essential for its proper functioning and resilience to disturbances.

- Symbiotic Relationship: The relationship between the gut microbiome and the human host is symbiotic, meaning both parties benefit from each other. The gut microbiota helps us digest certain foods, produces vitamins (e.g., B vitamins and vitamin K), and supports the development and function of the immune system.

- Gut-Brain Axis: The gut communicates with the brain through the gut-brain axis, a bidirectional communication system. This connection influences not only digestive health but also mental health and cognitive function.

- Immune Regulation: The gut microbiome plays a crucial role in regulating the immune system. A balanced gut microbiome can help prevent harmful pathogens from thriving and can reduce the risk of autoimmune diseases and allergies.

- Metabolic Function: The gut microbiome can influence metabolism, affecting how the body absorbs nutrients from food and how it stores and uses energy.

2.2 Factors Affecting Gut Health

Numerous factors can impact the composition and balance of the gut microbiome, influencing gut health. Some of the most significant factors include:

- Diet: A diet rich in fiber and diverse in plant-based foods promotes the growth of beneficial gut bacteria. On the other hand, diets high in processed foods, added sugars, and saturated fats can negatively impact gut health.

- Antibiotics and Medications: Antibiotics can disrupt the gut microbiome by indiscriminately killing both harmful and beneficial bacteria. Prolonged or frequent use of antibiotics can lead to imbalances in the gut microbiota.

- Stress: Chronic stress can alter gut motility, increase inflammation, and impact the diversity of the gut microbiome.

- Infections and Illnesses: Gastrointestinal infections can temporarily disturb the gut microbiome. Certain illnesses and conditions can also have long-term effects on gut health.

- Age: The gut microbiome evolves over a person's lifetime. Infants, for example, have a less diverse microbiome that becomes more complex as they age.

- Birth and Early Life: The method of birth (vaginal birth versus cesarean section) and feeding practices (breastfeeding versus formula feeding) can influence the

initial colonization of the gut
microbiome in infants.

- Physical Activity: Regular
physical activity may positively
influence gut health by supporting
a diverse gut microbiome.

- Environmental Exposures:
Environmental factors, such as
pollution and exposure to toxins,
can impact gut health indirectly.

- Probiotic and Prebiotic Intake:
Probiotics are live beneficial
microorganisms that can be
consumed through food or
supplements, while prebiotics are
non-digestible fibers that feed
beneficial gut bacteria. Both can
influence gut health positively.

2.3 Signs of an Imbalanced Gut Microbiome

An imbalanced gut microbiome, often referred to as dysbiosis, can manifest in various ways and may be associated with several health issues. Some signs of an imbalanced gut microbiome include:

1. Digestive Issues: These may include gas, bloating, diarrhea, constipation, and irritable bowel syndrome (IBS).

2. Weakened Immune Function: Frequent infections, allergies, or autoimmune conditions may be indicative of an imbalanced gut microbiome.

3. Mood and Mental Health Changes: An imbalanced gut microbiome

has been linked to mood swings, anxiety, depression, and cognitive issues.

4. Skin Conditions: Conditions like acne, eczema, and rosacea can sometimes be related to gut health.

5. Weight Fluctuations: Difficulty maintaining a healthy weight could be connected to gut microbiome imbalances.

6. Fatigue and Low Energy: Chronic fatigue and low energy levels may be associated with gut health issues.

It's important to note that these signs can be caused by various factors, and an imbalanced gut microbiome is just one of many potential contributors. If someone suspects gut health issues, it is recommended to consult with a healthcare professional who can conduct appropriate tests and provide personalized recommendations for improving gut health.

CHAPTER 3

Different Types of Probiotics

Probiotics are available in various strains, each with unique properties and potential health benefits. The most commonly studied and used probiotic strains fall into several categories, including Lactobacillus, Bifidobacterium, and other beneficial probiotic strains.

3.1 Lactobacillus Strains

Lactobacillus is a genus of probiotic bacteria that is naturally found in various fermented foods and dairy products. These bacteria are lactic acid producers, which means they convert sugars into lactic acid during fermentation. Lactobacillus strains are known for their ability to support digestive health and boost the immune system.

Some common Lactobacillus strains include:

- Lactobacillus acidophilus: Found in the human gut, mouth, and female reproductive tract, L. acidophilus is known for its ability to break down lactose (milk sugar) and produce lactase, making it beneficial for individuals with lactose intolerance. It may also support gut health and boost the immune system.

- Lactobacillus rhamnosus: This strain is well-studied for its potential to prevent and manage diarrhea, particularly antibiotic-associated diarrhea and infectious diarrhea. It may also help reduce the severity and duration of respiratory infections.

- Lactobacillus casei: L. casei is known for its immune-enhancing properties and its potential to alleviate symptoms of irritable bowel syndrome (IBS).

- Lactobacillus plantarum: This versatile strain is found in fermented foods and is known for its ability to survive the harsh conditions of the stomach and adhere to the intestinal lining. It may support gut health and reduce inflammation.

- Lactobacillus bulgaricus: Often used in the fermentation of yogurt, L. bulgaricus can help break down lactose and produce lactic acid. It may improve lactose digestion in lactose-intolerant individuals.

3.2 Bifidobacterium Strains

Bifidobacterium is another common genus of probiotic bacteria found in the human gastrointestinal tract. Bifidobacteria are essential for maintaining gut health, particularly in infants, and have been extensively studied for their beneficial effects on digestion and immunity.

Some common Bifidobacterium strains include:

- Bifidobacterium longum: This strain is one of the first probiotics to colonize the human gastrointestinal tract after birth. It may help with immune system development, reduce inflammation, and support gut health.

- Bifidobacterium bifidum: B. bifidum is known for its ability to compete with harmful bacteria and prevent their overgrowth in the gut. It may support gut health and improve the body's defense against infections.

- Bifidobacterium breve: B. breve is commonly found in breast milk and may contribute to the health of breastfed infants. It may also help alleviate symptoms of diarrhea and support gut health.

- Bifidobacterium lactis: This strain is often used in probiotic supplements and dairy products. B. lactis may improve digestive health, support the immune system, and help with lactose digestion.

3.3 Other Beneficial Probiotic Strains

Apart from Lactobacillus and Bifidobacterium strains, there are other probiotic strains that offer specific health benefits:

- Saccharomyces boulardii: Although technically a yeast, S. boulardii is considered a probiotic because it can support gut health by preventing the growth of harmful pathogens and reducing the severity of diarrhea, particularly in cases of antibiotic-associated diarrhea and infectious diarrhea.

- Streptococcus thermophilus: This probiotic strain is commonly used in the fermentation of yogurt and may support lactose digestion.

- Bacillus coagulans: This spore-forming probiotic has the ability to survive harsh conditions, such as those in the stomach, and can remain viable in food processing and storage. It may support gut health and immune function.

- Escherichia coli Nissle 1917: This specific strain of E. coli is non-pathogenic and can support gut health by promoting a balanced gut microbiome and reducing the growth of harmful bacteria.

Different strains of probiotics have varying effects, and not all strains will work for every individual or health condition. When considering probiotic supplementation, it's best to consult with a healthcare professional to determine which strains may be most appropriate for your specific health needs. Additionally, consuming a diverse range of probiotic-rich foods can also help support a healthy gut microbiome.

CHAPTER 4

Sources of Probiotics

Probiotics can be obtained from various sources, including fermented foods, probiotic supplements, and certain other products. Incorporating these sources into your diet can help promote a balanced gut microbiome and support overall health.

4.1 Fermented Foods

Fermented foods are natural sources of probiotics, as they contain live beneficial microorganisms that aid in the fermentation process. These foods undergo a controlled fermentation process, during which bacteria and yeasts convert sugars and carbohydrates into beneficial compounds like lactic acid and acetic acid. Some common fermented foods that provide probiotics include:

- Yogurt: Yogurt is made from milk fermented with specific strains of Lactobacillus and/or Bifidobacterium bacteria. Look for yogurt labeled as containing live and active cultures to ensure it provides probiotic benefits.

- Kefir: Kefir is a fermented dairy beverage made by adding kefir grains (a combination of bacteria and yeasts) to milk. It contains a broader range of probiotic strains compared to yogurt.

- Sauerkraut: Sauerkraut is fermented cabbage, traditionally made using only cabbage and salt. The fermentation process creates

probiotics and preserves the
cabbage.

- Kimchi: Kimchi is a Korean dish
  made from fermented vegetables,
  usually cabbage and radishes,
  seasoned with various spices. It is
  rich in probiotics and vitamins.

- Miso: Miso is a traditional
  Japanese seasoning made from
  fermented soybeans, rice, barley,
  or other grains. It is often used to
  make miso soup and adds probiotic
  benefits to the diet.

- Tempeh: Tempeh is a fermented
  soy product originating from
  Indonesia. It is made by
  fermenting soybeans, resulting in a
  firm, protein-rich product
  containing probiotics.

- Pickles (fermented, not vinegar-
  based): Traditional pickles are

made using the fermentation process rather than simply being pickled in vinegar. These types of pickles offer probiotic benefits.

- Natto: Natto is a traditional Japanese food made from fermented soybeans and contains the probiotic Bacillus subtilis.

Incorporating a variety of fermented foods into your diet can help increase the diversity of probiotic strains and support a healthy gut microbiome.

4.2 Probiotic Supplements

Probiotic supplements are commercially available in various forms, including capsules, tablets, powders, and liquids. These supplements contain concentrated amounts of specific probiotic strains, providing a convenient way to boost probiotic intake.

When choosing a probiotic supplement, consider the following factors:

- Strain Diversity: Look for a product that contains multiple strains of probiotics to provide a broader range of benefits.

- Colony Forming Units (CFUs): CFUs represent the number of viable microorganisms present in a probiotic product. Look for supplements with an appropriate CFU count, usually ranging from several billion to tens of billions per serving.

- Shelf Stability: Some probiotics require refrigeration to maintain their potency, while others are shelf-stable. Consider your lifestyle and storage options when selecting a product.

- Targeted Benefits: Some probiotic supplements are formulated to address specific health concerns, such as digestive issues, immune support, or women's health.

- Quality and Reputation: Choose products from reputable brands that undergo third-party testing to ensure quality and efficacy.

Always consult with a healthcare professional before starting any probiotic supplement, especially if you have specific health conditions or are taking medications.

4.3 Selecting the Right Probiotic Product

Choosing the right probiotic product can be a bit overwhelming given the vast array of options available. Here are some tips to help you select the most suitable probiotic for your needs:

1. Identify Your Health Goals: Determine what health benefits you seek from probiotics. Whether it's improving digestive health, boosting immunity, or addressing a specific condition, understanding your goals will guide your product selection.

2. Check the Strain Specifics: Look for products that list the specific probiotic strains and their respective benefits. Some strains are well-studied for particular

health benefits, so knowing the strains can help you make an informed decision.

3. Check CFU Count: Pay attention to the Colony Forming Units (CFUs) in the product. Higher CFUs don't necessarily mean better, as different strains require different quantities to be effective. Consider products with a CFU count ranging from several billion to tens of billions.

4. Consider Shelf Stability: If you prefer a product that doesn't require refrigeration or if you travel frequently, opt for shelf-stable probiotics. However, if you can store probiotics in the refrigerator without issues, refrigerated options may be more suitable.

5. Look for Quality Assurance:
    Choose products from reputable
    brands that conduct third-party
    testing to ensure the quality,
    potency, and safety of their
    probiotics.

6. Seek Professional Advice: If
    you're unsure which probiotic
    product is right for you, consult
    with a healthcare professional or a
    registered dictitian. They can
    provide personalized
    recommendations based on your
    health needs and medical history.

Individual responses to probiotics can
vary, and it may take some trial and
error to find the most beneficial
probiotic product for you.
Additionally, a balanced diet that
includes a variety of fermented foods

can complement probiotic supplementation and support a diverse gut microbiome.

CHAPTER 5

Incorporating Probiotics into Your Diet

Probiotics play a crucial role in maintaining a healthy gut microbiome, and incorporating them into your diet can have numerous benefits for your overall health. There are two main ways to add probiotics to your diet: through fermented foods and probiotic supplements. Here are some tips for incorporating both options into your daily routine:

5.1 Tips for Adding Fermented Foods to Your Meals

Fermented foods are a delicious and natural source of probiotics. Here's how you can include them in your meals:

1. Start with Yogurt: Yogurt is one of the most well-known probiotic-rich foods. Choose plain, unsweetened yogurt with live and active cultures. Add fresh fruits, nuts, or seeds for extra flavor and nutrients.

2. Experiment with Kefir: Kefir is a tangy and slightly effervescent fermented milk drink. It can be enjoyed on its own or used as a base for smoothies and salad dressings.

3. Savor Sauerkraut and Kimchi: Add sauerkraut or kimchi as a side dish or a topping to salads, sandwiches, or rice bowls. They add a burst of flavor and probiotic goodness.

4. Enjoy Miso Soup: Miso is a Japanese seasoning made from fermented soybeans. Use miso paste to make a delicious and nourishing miso soup with vegetables and tofu.

5. Make Your Own Pickles: Consider making homemade pickles using the fermentation method, which offers the added benefit of probiotics.

6. Include Tempeh in Your Meals: Tempeh is a versatile fermented soy product that can be used in various dishes like stir-fries, sandwiches, and salads.

7. Try Non-Dairy Options: If you are lactose intolerant or follow a dairy-free diet, explore non-dairy options like coconut kefir, soy yogurt, or almond milk yogurt with added probiotic cultures.

8. Ferment Your Own Foods: If you enjoy cooking, try fermenting vegetables, such as carrots, cucumbers, or beets, at home. Homemade fermented foods allow you to control the ingredients and fermentation process.

9. Be Mindful of Heat: Heat can destroy probiotics, so it's best to add fermented foods to dishes after cooking or at the end of the cooking process to preserve their probiotic content.

5.2 Integrating Probiotic Supplements into Your Routine

In addition to fermented foods, probiotic supplements can be a convenient way to boost your probiotic intake. Here's how to integrate them into your daily routine:

1. Consult with a Healthcare Professional: Before starting any probiotic supplement, consult with a healthcare professional or a registered dietitian to determine the right probiotic strains and dosages for your specific needs.

2. Choose High-Quality Supplements: Opt for probiotic supplements from reputable brands that provide detailed information about the strains, CFUs, and potential health benefits.

3. Follow Storage Recommendations:
    Follow the storage instructions on
    the supplement's packaging. Some
    probiotics require refrigeration to
    maintain their potency, while
    others are shelf-stable.

4. Take Probiotics with Food: Taking
    probiotics with meals may enhance
    their survival as the food provides
    a protective environment for the
    bacteria as they pass through the
    stomach.

5. Be Consistent: Incorporate
    probiotic supplements into your
    daily routine consistently to
    experience the potential benefits.
    Missing doses may reduce their
    effectiveness.

6. Consider Timing: Some people
    find it beneficial to take probiotics
    at specific times of the day, such

as before breakfast or before bedtime. Experiment and find what works best for you.

7. Monitor Your Response: Pay attention to how your body responds to probiotic supplementation. If you experience any adverse effects or if your health concerns persist, consult your healthcare provider for further guidance.

A diverse and balanced diet, including a variety of fermented foods and probiotic supplements, can contribute to a healthy gut microbiome. Additionally, lifestyle factors such as managing stress, staying physically active, and consuming a diet rich in fiber and whole foods also support overall gut health.

CHAPTER 6

Probiotics and Digestive Health

Probiotics play a significant role in supporting digestive health by promoting a balanced gut microbiome. They can help alleviate various digestive issues and improve overall gut function.

6.1 Alleviating Digestive Issues with Probiotics

Digestive issues can arise due to imbalances in the gut microbiome or disruptions in the gastrointestinal tract. Probiotics can help address these problems by:

1. Restoring Microbial Balance: Probiotics introduce beneficial bacteria to the gut, helping to restore a healthy balance of microorganisms. This balance is essential for proper digestion and the prevention of digestive discomfort.

2. Improving Nutrient Absorption: Probiotics aid in the breakdown of food particles, making nutrients more accessible for absorption by the body. This can enhance the efficiency of digestion and nutrient utilization.

3. Reducing Gut Inflammation: Probiotics may help reduce gut inflammation, which is often associated with conditions like irritable bowel syndrome (IBS) and inflammatory bowel disease (IBD).

4. Supporting Bowel Regularity: By promoting a balanced gut environment, probiotics can help regulate bowel movements and promote regularity.

5. Enhancing Gut Barrier Function: Probiotics contribute to maintaining a healthy gut barrier, preventing harmful substances from entering the bloodstream and reducing the risk of leaky gut syndrome.

6. Supporting Immune Function: A healthy gut microbiome is closely linked to a well-functioning immune system. Probiotics can bolster immune response and reduce the risk of infections that can affect the gastrointestinal tract.

6.2 Probiotics for Constipation and Diarrhea

Probiotics have shown promise in alleviating symptoms of both constipation and diarrhea, two common digestive issues that can significantly impact daily life.

Probiotics for Constipation:

- Bifidobacterium and Lactobacillus strains are among the most studied probiotics for constipation relief. They can help soften stools, improve transit time, and increase the frequency of bowel movements.

- Probiotics like Bifidobacterium animalis subsp. lactis DN-173 010 (also known as Bifidus Regularis) have been specifically studied for their potential to alleviate constipation and promote regular bowel movements.

- Probiotics can help modulate gut motility and increase the production of short-chain fatty acids, which can improve stool consistency and bowel movement regularity.

Probiotics for Diarrhea:

- Probiotics are known to be effective in managing different types of diarrhea, including antibiotic-associated diarrhea, infectious diarrhea, and traveler's diarrhea.

- Lactobacillus rhamnosus GG, Saccharomyces boulardii, and various Bifidobacterium strains are commonly studied probiotics for diarrhea relief.

- Probiotics work by competing with harmful pathogens for space and nutrients in the gut, producing antimicrobial substances, and stabilizing the gut barrier to prevent pathogens from causing diarrhea.

- Additionally, probiotics can help restore the gut microbiome after antibiotic use, reducing the risk of antibiotic-associated diarrhea.

It's important to note that not all probiotics are equally effective for every individual or every type of digestive issue. The benefits of probiotics may vary based on the specific strains used, the dosage, and an individual's unique gut microbiome composition. If you are experiencing persistent digestive issues, it's best to consult with a healthcare professional or a registered dietitian to determine the most appropriate probiotic strains and formulations for your needs. They can provide personalized recommendations to address your specific digestive health concerns.

6.3 Probiotics and Irritable Bowel Syndrome (IBS)

Probiotics have been extensively studied for their potential benefits in managing symptoms of Irritable Bowel Syndrome (IBS). IBS is a common gastrointestinal disorder characterized by chronic abdominal pain, bloating, and changes in bowel habits, such as diarrhea, constipation, or both. While the exact cause of IBS is not fully understood, imbalances in the gut microbiome and alterations in gut motility and sensitivity are believed to play a significant role.

Probiotics may offer several ways to help individuals with IBS:

1. Modulating Gut Microbiome: Probiotics can promote a healthier balance of gut bacteria, which may help reduce symptoms of IBS. Certain probiotic strains, such as Bifidobacterium and Lactobacillus, have shown promising results in clinical studies for managing IBS.

2. Reducing Inflammation: IBS is associated with low-grade inflammation in the gut. Probiotics can have anti-inflammatory effects, which may help alleviate gut inflammation and reduce symptoms.

3. Alleviating Bloating and Gas: Probiotics can improve the

digestion of certain carbohydrates, reducing the production of gas in the gut, which can contribute to bloating and discomfort in individuals with IBS.

4. Normalizing Bowel Movements: Some probiotics can help regulate bowel movements by influencing gut motility, leading to more consistent and less erratic bowel habits.

5. Relieving Abdominal Pain: Probiotics may reduce the perception of pain in the gut and provide relief from abdominal discomfort in individuals with IBS.

Several probiotic strains have been studied for their potential benefits in managing IBS, including:

- Bifidobacterium infantis: This strain has shown promising results in improving abdominal pain and bloating in individuals with IBS.

- Lactobacillus plantarum: Studies have suggested that L. plantarum may reduce IBS symptoms, particularly in terms of bloating and bowel movement irregularities.

- Bifidobacterium breve: This strain has shown positive effects in reducing bloating and improving bowel movements in individuals with IBS.

- Lactobacillus acidophilus: L. acidophilus has been studied for its potential to improve gut transit time and reduce symptoms in IBS patients.

It's essential to note that the effectiveness of probiotics in managing IBS can vary between individuals, and not all strains will work for everyone. Additionally, the optimal dosage and duration of probiotic use for IBS management are still subjects of ongoing research.

If you have IBS and are considering using probiotics as part of your management plan, it's crucial to consult with a healthcare professional or a registered dietitian. They can help you choose the most suitable probiotic strains, recommend appropriate dosages, and provide guidance on integrating probiotics into your IBS management plan alongside other lifestyle and dietary interventions

CHAPTER 7

Probiotics and Immune System Support

7.1 The Connection Between Probiotics and Immunity

The gut and the immune system are closely interconnected. Approximately 70-80% of the body's immune cells reside in the gut-associated lymphoid tissue (GALT). This complex relationship between the gut and the immune system is referred to as the gut-immune axis.

Probiotics, by promoting a balanced and diverse gut microbiome, can influence the gut-immune axis and enhance immune system function. A well-functioning gut microbiome helps support the immune system in several ways:

1. Regulation of Immune Response: Probiotics can help regulate the immune system's response to pathogens and antigens. They can promote a balanced immune response, preventing unnecessary inflammation and reducing the risk of autoimmune reactions.

2. Pathogen Exclusion: Probiotics compete with harmful bacteria and pathogens for space and nutrients in the gut, preventing their overgrowth. This exclusion of pathogens can reduce the risk of infections and support the immune

system's ability to defend against invaders.

3. Production of Beneficial Compounds: Some probiotic strains can produce beneficial compounds, such as short-chain fatty acids (SCFAs), which have anti-inflammatory properties and support immune health.

4. Maintenance of Gut Barrier: Probiotics contribute to maintaining the integrity of the gut barrier. A strong gut barrier prevents harmful substances and pathogens from entering the bloodstream and causing immune responses.

7.2 Enhancing Immune Function with Probiotics

Probiotics have been studied for their potential to enhance immune function and provide immune system support. Some ways probiotics can boost immunity include:

1. Reducing the Severity and Duration of Infections: Probiotics, especially strains like Lactobacillus and Bifidobacterium, have been associated with reduced severity and duration of common infections like the common cold and respiratory tract infections.

2. Supporting Respiratory Health: Probiotics may help reduce the risk of upper respiratory tract infections and improve respiratory symptoms.

3. Immune Support in Infants and
   Children: Probiotics can play a
   role in supporting the developing
   immune system in infants and
   young children. Certain probiotic
   strains have been studied for their
   potential to reduce the risk of
   infections in this population.

4. Managing Allergic Reactions:
   Probiotics have been investigated
   for their role in modulating the
   immune response and reducing the
   severity of allergic reactions, such
   as allergic rhinitis and eczema.

5. Immune Support during Stress:
   Probiotics may help mitigate the
   negative impact of chronic stress
   on the immune system, promoting
   a balanced immune response.

It's essential to note that the immune-
boosting effects of probiotics can vary

between individuals and depend on factors such as the specific strains used, the dosage, and an individual's overall health and immune status. Additionally, the effectiveness of probiotics in providing immune system support may vary depending on the strain's ability to survive stomach acid and reach the gut alive.

If you are considering using probiotics to support your immune system, it's best to consult with a healthcare professional or a registered dietitian. They can help you choose the most suitable probiotic strains based on your specific health needs and provide recommendations on dosage and duration of use. Probiotics can be a valuable addition to a comprehensive approach to overall health and immunity, alongside a balanced diet, regular physical activity, adequate sleep, and other healthy lifestyle practices.

CHAPTER 8
Probiotics and Mental Health

8.1 The Gut-Brain Axis: Understanding the Connection

The gut-brain axis is a complex bidirectional communication system that connects the gut (specifically, the gut microbiome) to the brain. This connection involves neural, hormonal, and immune pathways that allow constant communication between the two organs. The gut and the brain are linked through the vagus nerve and various signaling molecules.

The gut microbiome plays a crucial role in this communication. The diverse community of microorganisms in the gut produces various metabolites, neurotransmitters, and other bioactive compounds that can influence brain function and mental health. Some of these compounds, such as serotonin and gamma-aminobutyric acid (GABA), are neurotransmitters that play vital roles in mood regulation and emotional well-being.

Factors that can influence the gut-brain axis and impact mental health include:

1. Gut Microbiome Composition: The balance of beneficial and harmful bacteria in the gut can influence the production of neurotransmitters and other

compounds that affect mood and cognitive function.

2. Gut Permeability: An imbalanced gut microbiome and gut inflammation can lead to increased gut permeability (leaky gut), allowing harmful substances to enter the bloodstream and potentially impact brain function.

3. Immune System Activation: Gut inflammation and imbalances in the gut microbiome can trigger immune responses that may affect brain function and contribute to mental health issues.

4. Neurotransmitter Production: The gut microbiome can influence the production and metabolism of neurotransmitters in the gut and in the brain.

8.2 Probiotics for Reducing Anxiety and Depression

Research into the potential benefits of probiotics for mental health, specifically anxiety and depression, is a rapidly growing area of interest. Some studies have suggested that certain probiotic strains may have a positive impact on reducing anxiety and depression symptoms. Here are some ways in which probiotics may potentially benefit mental health:

1. Serotonin Production: Certain probiotics can influence the production of serotonin, a neurotransmitter that plays a key role in mood regulation. Higher serotonin levels are associated with improved mood and reduced anxiety.

2. Inflammation Reduction:
    Probiotics may help reduce gut
    inflammation, which can have
    indirect effects on brain health.
    Chronic inflammation has been
    linked to an increased risk of
    anxiety and depression.

3. Communication via the Gut-Brain
    Axis: Probiotics can communicate
    with the brain through the gut-
    brain axis, potentially influencing
    brain function and emotional well-
    being.

4. Stress Response Regulation: Some
    probiotics have been studied for
    their potential to modulate the
    body's stress response, leading to
    reduced anxiety levels.

While the research on probiotics and
mental health is promising, it's
essential to note that the effects of

probiotics on anxiety and depression can vary between individuals. The optimal probiotic strains, dosages, and treatment duration for mental health support are still subjects of ongoing research.

If you are considering using probiotics to support mental health, it's essential to consult with a healthcare professional or a mental health specialist. They can provide guidance on which probiotic strains may be most suitable for your specific needs and can work with you to develop a comprehensive approach to mental health that may include probiotics alongside other therapeutic interventions, such as counseling or psychotherapy. Probiotics can be a valuable addition to a holistic approach to mental well-being, but

they are not a substitute for
professional mental health care when
needed.

CHAPTER 9

Probiotics for Women's Health

9.1 Probiotics and Vaginal Health

The vaginal microbiome plays a critical role in maintaining women's urogenital health. A balanced vaginal microbiome consists of various beneficial bacteria, primarily dominated by Lactobacillus species. These bacteria help maintain the vaginal pH, produce lactic acid, and create a hostile environment for harmful pathogens, reducing the risk of infections.

Probiotics can support vaginal health by:

1. Restoring and Maintaining a Balanced Vaginal Microbiome: Probiotic strains, especially Lactobacillus species like Lactobacillus crispatus, Lactobacillus rhamnosus, and Lactobacillus reuteri, can be beneficial in promoting a balanced vaginal microbiome.

2. Preventing and Managing Vaginal Infections: Probiotics can help prevent and manage common vaginal infections, such as bacterial vaginosis and yeast infections (e.g., candidiasis).

3. Supporting Urinary Tract Health: Probiotics may also have some benefits for urinary tract health,

helping reduce the risk of urinary tract infections (UTIs).

When considering probiotics for vaginal health, it's essential to use products specifically formulated for vaginal use. Probiotic vaginal suppositories, capsules, or creams are available that contain strains specifically targeted for vaginal health. As always, it's best to consult with a healthcare professional before using any new products, especially if you have a history of recurrent vaginal infections or other gynecological issues.

9.2 Probiotics during Pregnancy and Breastfeeding

Probiotics can also be beneficial during pregnancy and breastfeeding. The gut microbiome of pregnant women and breastfeeding mothers can influence their health as well as the health of their infants. Here are some potential benefits of probiotics during this period:

1. Supporting Maternal Gut Health: Pregnancy and breastfeeding can lead to changes in gut microbiota composition. Probiotics can help maintain a balanced gut microbiome, supporting maternal digestive health.

2. Reducing the Risk of Gestational Diabetes: Some studies suggest that certain probiotic strains may

help reduce the risk of gestational diabetes, a condition that develops during pregnancy.

3. Immune Support: Probiotics can support the maternal immune system during pregnancy and breastfeeding, which is important for both the mother and the developing baby.

4. Reducing the Risk of Allergies: There is some evidence to suggest that probiotic supplementation during pregnancy and breastfeeding may help reduce the risk of allergic conditions in infants.

When considering probiotics during pregnancy and breastfeeding, it's essential to choose products that are safe for use during this sensitive period. Look for probiotics with strains that have been well-studied and are generally recognized as safe for pregnancy and breastfeeding. Always consult with a healthcare professional before taking any supplements, including probiotics, during pregnancy or while breastfeeding, to ensure they are appropriate for your individual health needs.

Probiotics can be a valuable addition to a comprehensive approach to women's health, promoting vaginal and gut health and supporting overall well-being during pregnancy and breastfeeding. However, individual responses to probiotics may vary, and it's best to work with a healthcare professional to determine the most suitable probiotic strains and dosages for your specific health concerns.

CHAPTER 10

Prebiotics: The Fuel for Probiotics

10.1 What are Prebiotics?

Prebiotics are a type of dietary fiber that serves as food for probiotics, the beneficial bacteria residing in the gut. Unlike probiotics, which are live microorganisms, prebiotics are non-living compounds that pass through the upper gastrointestinal tract undigested. They reach the colon, where they are selectively fermented by beneficial gut bacteria, providing them with nourishment and allowing them to thrive.

The primary role of prebiotics is to support the growth and activity of probiotics, promoting a healthy and diverse gut microbiome. They contribute to overall gut health and play a vital role in maintaining the balance of the gut ecosystem.

Common examples of prebiotics include:

1. Inulin: Found in foods like chicory root, Jerusalem artichokes, and onions.

2. Fructooligosaccharides (FOS): Present in foods such as bananas, garlic, and asparagus.

3. Galactooligosaccharides (GOS): Found in human breast milk and some dairy products.

4. Oligofructose: Found in foods like leeks, asparagus, and wheat.

Prebiotics are not affected by heat or stomach acid, making them relatively stable and suitable for various cooking and food processing methods.

10.2 Combining Probiotics and Prebiotics for Optimal Results

The combination of probiotics and prebiotics is known as synbiotics. Synbiotics work synergistically to improve gut health and support overall well-being. Here's how combining probiotics and prebiotics can lead to optimal results:

1. Enhancing Probiotic Viability: Prebiotics act as a source of nourishment for probiotics, helping them survive and thrive in the gut. When taken together,

prebiotics can increase the survival rate of probiotics through the harsh acidic environment of the stomach and facilitate their colonization in the gut.

2. Promoting Beneficial Microbial Growth: Prebiotics selectively stimulate the growth and activity of beneficial probiotic bacteria. By providing specific nutrients, prebiotics support the growth of these beneficial bacteria, helping them dominate the gut microbiome.

3. Strengthening the Gut Barrier: A balanced gut microbiome promoted by synbiotics helps strengthen the gut barrier, reducing the risk of leaky gut and related health issues.

4. Supporting Digestive Health: Synbiotics have been shown to have positive effects on digestive health, alleviating symptoms of gastrointestinal disorders like irritable bowel syndrome (IBS) and constipation.

5. Boosting Immune Function: A healthy gut microbiome supported by synbiotics can enhance the immune system's function, improving the body's ability to defend against infections and harmful pathogens.

6. Potentiating Health Benefits: The combination of probiotics and prebiotics may potentiate their individual health benefits, resulting in greater overall improvements in gut health and well-being.

Synbiotic-rich foods and supplements are available in the market. When choosing synbiotic products, look for a combination of well-researched probiotic strains and prebiotics with known health benefits. Additionally, consider consulting with a healthcare professional or a registered dietitian to determine the most suitable synbiotic regimen based on your specific health needs and medical history.

Overall, incorporating prebiotics into your diet alongside probiotics can be a proactive approach to supporting gut health and maintaining a thriving gut microbiome. By fostering a diverse and balanced gut ecosystem, synbiotics can contribute to overall health and well-being.

CHAPTER 11

Safety and Side Effects of Probiotics

11.1 Potential Side Effects of Probiotic Use

Probiotics are generally considered safe for most healthy individuals when taken as recommended. However, some people may experience mild side effects, especially during the initial days of probiotic supplementation. Common side effects include:

1. Digestive Upset: Some individuals may experience mild digestive issues such as gas, bloating, or an increase in bowel movements

when starting probiotics. These symptoms often subside as the gut microbiome adjusts to the new probiotic strains.

2. Allergic Reactions: In rare cases, people may be allergic to specific probiotic strains or components in probiotic products. Allergic reactions can manifest as hives, itching, or difficulty breathing. If you experience any severe allergic symptoms, discontinue use and seek medical attention immediately.

3. Infection in Certain Populations: In extremely rare cases, particularly in individuals with compromised immune systems or underlying health conditions, probiotics may cause serious infections. However, such cases are exceptionally uncommon.

It's essential to note that the vast majority of people tolerate probiotics well, and side effects, when they occur, are generally mild and transient. If you experience persistent or severe side effects, stop using the probiotic and consult with a healthcare professional.

When choosing a probiotic product, consider the strain, CFU count, and the quality of the brand. Probiotics from reputable manufacturers undergo rigorous testing to ensure safety and efficacy.

11.2 Probiotics for Individuals with Weakened Immune Systems

For individuals with weakened immune systems, such as those undergoing chemotherapy, organ transplant recipients, or those with immune disorders, the use of probiotics requires extra caution. The gut microbiome plays a crucial role in immune system modulation, and introducing live microorganisms can have unpredictable effects in individuals with compromised immune function.

While some research has shown potential benefits of probiotics in certain immune-related conditions, the safety of probiotics in immunocompromised individuals remains a concern. Probiotic supplementation in these populations should only be undertaken under the guidance and close supervision of a healthcare professional.

Individuals with weakened immune systems are at a higher risk of probiotic-associated infections, including bloodstream infections. The risk of these infections may be more significant in individuals with central venous catheters or recent surgical procedures.

If you have a weakened immune system or a chronic health condition, consult with your healthcare provider before starting any probiotic supplementation. They can assess your individual health status and help determine if probiotics are safe and appropriate for you. In some cases, probiotics may be recommended as part of a comprehensive treatment plan, while in others, their use may be contraindicated.

Ultimately, the safety of probiotics largely depends on the individual's health status and the specific probiotic strains used. It is always wise to seek personalized advice from a healthcare professional to ensure that probiotics are suitable for your particular circumstances.

CHAPTER 12

Incorporating Probiotic Lifestyle Habits

12.1 Lifestyle Factors that Support Probiotic Health

In addition to incorporating probiotic-rich foods and supplements, several lifestyle factors can positively influence probiotic health and overall gut well-being. Here are some lifestyle habits that support a healthy gut microbiome:

1. Balanced Diet: Consume a diverse and balanced diet rich in fruits,

vegetables, whole grains, and sources of healthy fats and proteins. A diverse diet provides essential nutrients to support the growth and activity of beneficial gut bacteria.

2. High-Fiber Foods: Include plenty of high-fiber foods in your diet, such as legumes, whole grains, nuts, seeds, fruits, and vegetables. Fiber serves as a prebiotic, feeding beneficial gut bacteria and promoting a healthy gut microbiome.

3. Avoid Excessive Sugar and Processed Foods: Limit the consumption of sugary and processed foods, as they can disrupt the balance of gut bacteria and promote the growth of harmful microbes.

4. Stay Hydrated: Drink plenty of water to support digestion and keep the gut hydrated.

5. Regular Exercise: Engage in regular physical activity, as exercise has been associated with positive effects on gut health. Exercise may help enhance gut motility and promote a diverse gut microbiome.

6. Manage Stress: Chronic stress can negatively impact gut health and the gut-brain axis. Practice stress-reducing techniques like meditation, deep breathing, yoga, or spending time in nature.

7. Avoid Overuse of Antibiotics: Use antibiotics only when prescribed by a healthcare professional, and avoid unnecessary use. Antibiotics

can disrupt the gut microbiome, leading to imbalances.

8. Get Enough Sleep: Prioritize good sleep hygiene to support overall health, including gut health. Aim for 7-9 hours of quality sleep per night.

9. Limit Alcohol and Smoking: Excessive alcohol consumption and smoking can negatively impact the gut microbiome. Limit these habits for better gut health.

10. Avoid Unnecessary Antibacterial Products: Overuse of antibacterial products can disrupt the natural balance of bacteria on the skin and in the gut. Use these products sparingly and only when necessary.

12.2 Balancing Diet, Exercise, and Probiotics

A well-rounded approach to gut health involves balancing diet, exercise, and probiotics:

1. Diet: Consume a diet rich in probiotic and prebiotic foods to support beneficial gut bacteria. Incorporate fermented foods like yogurt, kefir, sauerkraut, kimchi, and tempeh into your meals. Also, include high-fiber foods like fruits, vegetables, whole grains, and legumes to feed the gut microbiome.

2. Probiotic Supplements: If you cannot consume enough probiotic-rich foods, consider probiotic supplements. Choose high-quality supplements with specific strains that target your health concerns,

and follow the recommended
dosage.

3. Exercise: Engage in regular
   physical activity to support gut
   motility and overall gut health.
   Aim for a mix of cardiovascular
   exercises, strength training, and
   flexibility exercises.

4. Stress Management: Practice
   stress-reducing techniques to
   minimize the negative impact of
   stress on gut health. Mindfulness
   practices like meditation or yoga
   can be helpful.

5. Hydration: Stay hydrated by
   drinking enough water throughout
   the day. Proper hydration is
   essential for overall digestive
   health.

6. Balanced Lifestyle: Maintain a
   balanced lifestyle that includes

sufficient sleep, regular mealtimes, and time for relaxation and enjoyment.

Individual responses to lifestyle changes and probiotic supplementation may vary. If you have specific health concerns or medical conditions, consult with a healthcare professional or a registered dietitian to develop a personalized plan that suits your needs. By incorporating these lifestyle habits and fostering a balanced gut microbiome, you can support your overall health and well-being.

CHAPTER 13

Embracing Probiotics for a Healthier Future

Probiotics offer a promising path towards a healthier future by promoting gut health and supporting overall well-being. As our understanding of the gut microbiome grows, the importance of probiotics in maintaining a balanced and diverse gut ecosystem becomes increasingly evident. Here are some reasons why embracing probiotics can contribute to a healthier future:

1. Gut Health Optimization: Probiotics play a crucial role in

promoting gut health by restoring and maintaining a balanced gut microbiome. A healthy gut is linked to improved digestion, better nutrient absorption, and reduced gastrointestinal issues.

2. Enhanced Immune Function: A thriving gut microbiome supports a well-functioning immune system. By incorporating probiotics, we can bolster our body's defense against infections and pathogens, contributing to overall immune health.

3. Mental Well-being: The gut-brain axis highlights the bidirectional communication between the gut and the brain. Probiotics have the potential to positively influence mental health by supporting a healthy gut microbiome, which can

impact mood and emotional well-being.

4. Disease Prevention: Probiotics have shown promise in preventing and managing certain health conditions, including gastrointestinal disorders, allergies, and even metabolic conditions like diabetes.

5. Antibiotic Support: Probiotics can be beneficial during and after antibiotic treatment to counteract the disruption of beneficial gut bacteria caused by antibiotics.

6. Women's Health: Probiotics can support vaginal health and the prevention of vaginal infections, contributing to improved women's health.

7. Promoting Longevity: A healthy gut microbiome has been

associated with longevity and healthy aging. By nurturing our gut with probiotics, we can strive for a longer, healthier life.

8. Sustainable Health Approach: Probiotics are a natural and sustainable approach to supporting health. Incorporating probiotic-rich foods into our diet and using high-quality probiotic supplements aligns with a holistic approach to well-being.

9. Personalized Health: As research advances, we are learning more about the personalized nature of gut health. Embracing probiotics allows individuals to explore and tailor their gut health to their unique needs.

10. Potential Future Discoveries: The field of gut microbiome research is continually evolving, and ongoing research may uncover even more benefits and applications of probiotics in various aspects of health.

As we look forward to a healthier future, embracing probiotics as a part of our daily lives can be a proactive step towards maintaining optimal gut health and overall well-being. By adopting a well-rounded approach that includes a balanced diet, regular exercise, stress management, and the use of probiotics, we can empower ourselves to take charge of our health and lay the foundation for a brighter and healthier future. As with any health-related decisions, consulting with healthcare professionals and

registered dietitians can provide
personalized guidance and support on
incorporating probiotics into your
health journey.

www.ingramcontent.com/pod-product-compliance
Lightning Source LLC
Chambersburg PA
CBHW071607270726
48661CB00019B/1639